PRE DIABETES VEGETARIAN MEAL PLAN FOR BEGINNERS

Easy and Delicious Plant-Based Recipes and Meal Plans to Prevent and Manage Prediabetes, Perfect for Beginners Starting a Healthy Vegetarian Lifestyle

By Mia Bennett

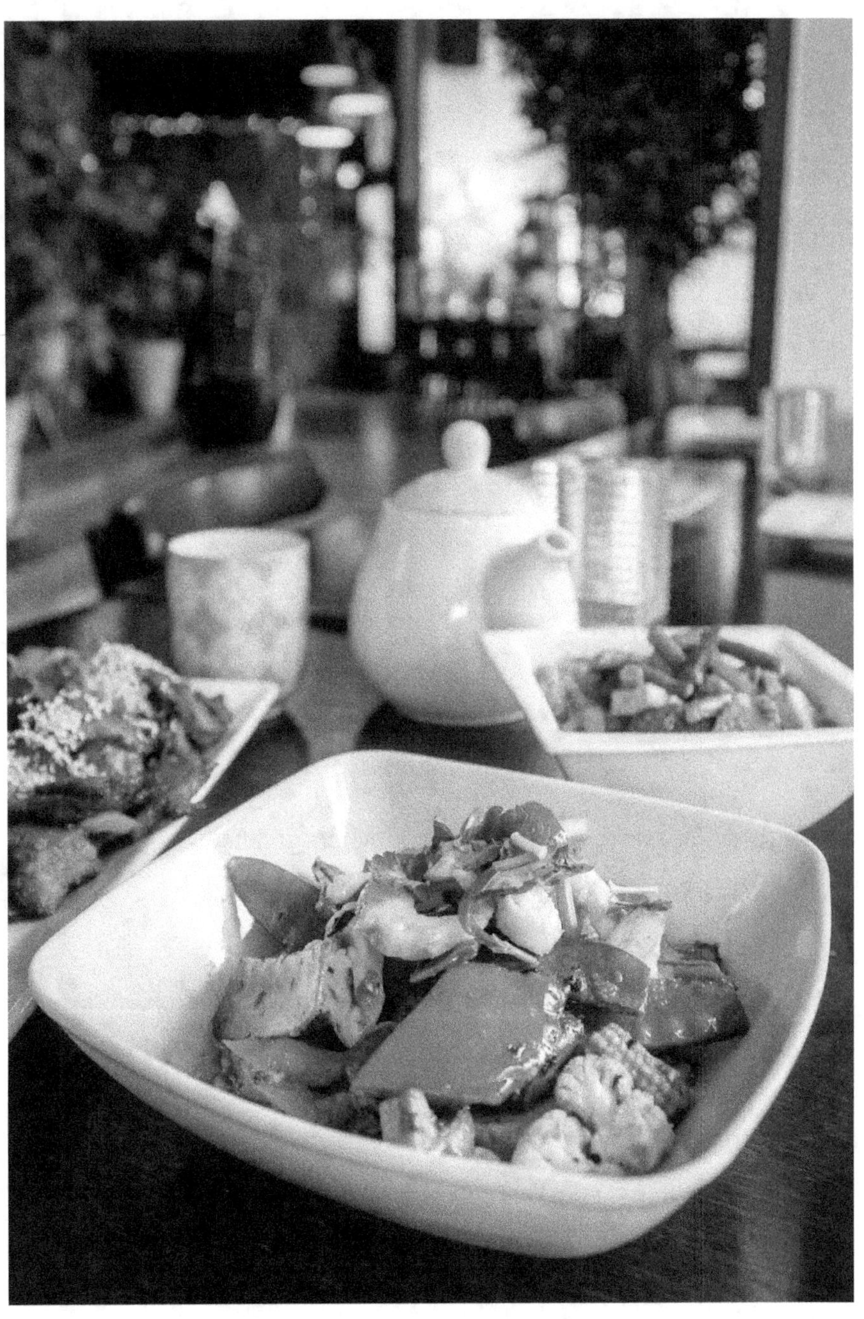

TABLE OF CONTENTS

Chapter 5: Snacks and Appetizers 80

INTRODUCTION

Prediabetes – the state where your blood sugar is higher than normal but not quite high enough for a type 2 diabetes diagnosis – can feel like a crossroads. It's a wake-up call to take action and prevent the progression of the disease. This is where a well-constructed vegetarian diet shines. Let's delve into prediabetes, explore the advantages of a plant-based approach, and equip you with the knowledge to craft delicious and effective meals.

Understanding Prediabetes: The Lowdown

Imagine your body is a grand estate, and blood sugar is the currency used to fuel its functions. In prediabetes, the gates controlling this currency flow become sluggish. The body produces insulin, the key that unlocks cells to absorb sugar, but it's not as effective as it should be. This leads to excess sugar circulating in the bloodstream, a condition that can pave the way for type 2 diabetes if left unchecked.

Why Go Vegetarian for Prediabetes? A Boon for Blood Sugar Balance

A vegetarian diet, rich in fruits, vegetables, whole grains, legumes, nuts, and seeds, offers a treasure trove of benefits for prediabetes management. Here's how:

- **Fiber Powerhouse:** Plant-based meals are naturally high in fiber, which slows down sugar absorption, preventing those blood sugar spikes.
- **Weight Management:** Maintaining a healthy weight is crucial for prediabetes. Vegetarian diets tend to be lower in calories and fat, promoting weight loss or healthy weight management.
- **Nutrient Richness:** Think vibrant vegetables packed with antioxidants, legumes brimming with protein and complex carbs, and nuts and seeds bursting with healthy fats. These provide essential nutrients for overall well-being.

Essential Ingredients and Nutrients: Your Vegetarian Arsenal

Now, let's stock your kitchen with the building blocks of healthy prediabetic meals:

- **Non-Starchy Vegetables:** Leafy greens, broccoli, cauliflower – these are your low-carb, high-fiber champions.

- **Starchy Vegetables:** Sweet potatoes, corn, peas – enjoy these in moderation for sustained energy.

- **Whole Grains:** Brown rice, quinoa, whole-wheat bread – choose these complex carbs over refined grains.

- **Legumes:** Beans, lentils – a vegetarian's protein powerhouse, loaded with fiber too.

- **Healthy Fats:** Avocados, nuts, seeds – essential for satiety and heart health.

- **Healthy Oils:** Olive oil, canola oil – use these sparingly for cooking.

Planning and Prepping: Effortless Vegetarian Meals

Conquering prediabetes doesn't have to mean hours in the kitchen. Here are some tips for meal planning and prep:

- **Batch Cooking:** Cook a large pot of lentil soup or a veggie stir-fry on the weekend for easy meals throughout the week.

- **Prep is Key:** Wash and chop vegetables beforehand for quick and healthy snacking or salad building.

- **Embrace Meatless Mondays:** Start by incorporating one vegetarian day a week, gradually increasing as you get comfortable.
- **Seasoning is Magic:** Explore herbs and spices to add depth of flavor to your vegetarian dishes.

Remember, this is a journey, not a sprint. By understanding prediabetes, embracing the power of a plant-based diet, and incorporating these tips, you can create a delicious path towards a healthier you. Don't hesitate to consult a registered dietitian for personalized guidance. With the right approach, you can turn this into an empowering opportunity to take charge of your health and well-being.

Chapter 1: 30 Day Meal Plan

Week 1

Day 1

- Breakfast: Avocado Toast with Tomatoes and Microgreens
- Lunch: Lentil Salad with Feta and Spinach
- Dinner: Stuffed Bell Peppers with Quinoa and Vegetables
- Snack: Hummus with Carrot and Cucumber Sticks
- Dessert: Chia Seed Pudding with Mixed Berries

Day 2

- Breakfast: Quinoa Breakfast Bowl with Berries and Almonds
- Lunch: Chickpea and Avocado Sandwich
- Dinner: Eggplant Parmesan with Whole Wheat Pasta
- Snack: Baked Kale Chips
- Dessert: Dark Chocolate Avocado Mousse

Day 3

- Breakfast: Greek Yogurt with Chia Seeds and Fresh Fruit
- Lunch: Quinoa Salad with Roasted Vegetables
- Dinner: Veggie Burger with Sweet Potato Fries
- Snack: Edamame with Sea Salt

- Dessert: Baked Apples with Cinnamon

Day 4

- Breakfast: Spinach and Mushroom Frittata
- Lunch: Vegetable Stir-Fry with Tofu
- Dinner: Spaghetti Squash with Marinara Sauce
- Snack: Stuffed Mini Peppers with Goat Cheese
- Dessert: Banana Ice Cream with Almond Butter

Day 5

- Breakfast: Overnight Oats with Flaxseeds and Blueberries
- Lunch: Caprese Salad with Balsamic Glaze
- Dinner: Lentil and Vegetable Stew
- Snack: Avocado and Black Bean Salsa
- Dessert: Carrot Cake Bites

Day 6

- Breakfast: Whole Grain Pancakes with Fresh Strawberries
- Lunch: Mediterranean Chickpea Bowl
- Dinner: Cauliflower Pizza with Fresh Tomatoes and Basil
- Snack: Greek Yogurt with Fresh Fruit and Nuts
- Dessert: Mixed Berry Crumble

Day 7

- Breakfast: Smoothie Bowl with Nuts and Seeds
- Lunch: Black Bean and Corn Salad
- Dinner: Zucchini Noodles with Avocado Pesto
- Snack: Spicy Roasted Chickpeas
- Dessert: Coconut Macaroons

Week 2

Day 8

- Breakfast: Scrambled Tofu with Veggies
- Lunch: Veggie Wrap with Hummus and Sprouts
- Dinner: Baked Falafel with Tzatziki
- Snack: Veggie Spring Rolls with Peanut Sauce
- Dessert: Vegan Chocolate Chip Cookies

Day 9

- Breakfast: Sweet Potato Hash with Black Beans
- Lunch: Greek Salad with Olives and Cucumber
- Dinner: Spinach and Ricotta Stuffed Shells
- Snack: Caprese Skewers
- Dessert: Fresh Fruit Salad with Mint

Day 10

- Breakfast: Oatmeal with Apple Slices and Cinnamon
- Lunch: Sweet Potato and Black Bean Tacos
- Dinner: Mushroom and Spinach Risotto
- Snack: Guacamole with Whole Grain Tortilla Chips
- Dessert: Mango Sorbet

Day 11

- Breakfast: Buckwheat Porridge with Banana and Walnuts
- Lunch: Cauliflower Rice with Pesto
- Dinner: Roasted Vegetable Tacos
- Snack: Cottage Cheese with Pineapple
- Dessert: Peanut Butter and Banana Bites

Day 12

- Breakfast: Multigrain Muffins with Zucchini
- Lunch: Spinach and Strawberry Salad with Walnuts
- Dinner: Broccoli and Tofu Stir-Fry
- Snack: Almond Butter on Whole Grain Crackers
- Dessert: Roasted Pears with Honey

Day 13

- Breakfast: Breakfast Burrito with Avocado and Salsa
- Lunch: Edamame and Kale Salad

- Dinner: Chickpea and Spinach Curry
- Snack: Celery Sticks with Peanut Butter
- Dessert: Raw Date and Nut Bars

Day 14

- Breakfast: Chia Pudding with Coconut Milk and Mango
- Lunch: Roasted Beet and Goat Cheese Salad
- Dinner: Ratatouille with Brown Rice
- Snack: Mini Veggie Frittatas
- Dessert: Lemon Blueberry Muffins

Week 3

Day 15

- Breakfast: Whole Wheat Bagel with Hummus and Cucumber
- Lunch: Vegan Sushi Rolls with Avocado and Cucumber
- Dinner: Vegan Shepherd's Pie
- Snack: Roasted Pumpkin Seeds
- Dessert: Apple Cinnamon Oatmeal Bars

Day 16

- Breakfast: Avocado Toast with Tomatoes and Microgreens
- Lunch: Lentil Salad with Feta and Spinach

- Dinner: Stuffed Bell Peppers with Quinoa and Vegetables

- Snack: Hummus with Carrot and Cucumber Sticks

- Dessert: Chia Seed Pudding with Mixed Berries

Day 17

- Breakfast: Quinoa Breakfast Bowl with Berries and Almonds

- Lunch: Chickpea and Avocado Sandwich

- Dinner: Eggplant Parmesan with Whole Wheat Pasta

- Snack: Baked Kale Chips

- Dessert: Dark Chocolate Avocado Mousse

Day 18

- Breakfast: Greek Yogurt with Chia Seeds and Fresh Fruit

- Lunch: Quinoa Salad with Roasted Vegetables

- Dinner: Veggie Burger with Sweet Potato Fries

- Snack: Edamame with Sea Salt

- Dessert: Baked Apples with Cinnamon

Day 19

- Breakfast: Spinach and Mushroom Frittata

- Lunch: Vegetable Stir-Fry with Tofu

- Dinner: Spaghetti Squash with Marinara Sauce

- Snack: Stuffed Mini Peppers with Goat Cheese

- Dessert: Banana Ice Cream with Almond Butter

Day 20

- Breakfast: Overnight Oats with Flaxseeds and Blueberries
- Lunch: Caprese Salad with Balsamic Glaze
- Dinner: Lentil and Vegetable Stew
- Snack: Avocado and Black Bean Salsa
- Dessert: Carrot Cake Bites

Day 21

- Breakfast: Whole Grain Pancakes with Fresh Strawberries
- Lunch: Mediterranean Chickpea Bowl
- Dinner: Cauliflower Pizza with Fresh Tomatoes and Basil
- Snack: Greek Yogurt with Fresh Fruit and Nuts
- Dessert: Mixed Berry Crumble

Week 4

Day 22

- Breakfast: Smoothie Bowl with Nuts and Seeds
- Lunch: Black Bean and Corn Salad
- Dinner: Zucchini Noodles with Avocado Pesto
- Snack: Spicy Roasted Chickpeas
- Dessert: Coconut Macaroons

Day 23

- Breakfast: Scrambled Tofu with Veggies
- Lunch: Veggie Wrap with Hummus and Sprouts
- Dinner: Baked Falafel with Tzatziki
- Snack: Veggie Spring Rolls with Peanut Sauce
- Dessert: Vegan Chocolate Chip Cookies

Day 24

- Breakfast: Sweet Potato Hash with Black Beans
- Lunch: Greek Salad with Olives and Cucumber
- Dinner: Spinach and Ricotta Stuffed Shells
- Snack: Caprese Skewers
- Dessert: Fresh Fruit Salad with Mint

Day 25

- Breakfast: Oatmeal with Apple Slices and Cinnamon
- Lunch: Sweet Potato and Black Bean Tacos
- Dinner: Mushroom and Spinach Risotto
- Snack: Guacamole with Whole Grain Tortilla Chips
- Dessert: Mango Sorbet

Day 26

- Breakfast: Buckwheat Porridge with Banana and Walnuts
- Lunch: Cauliflower Rice with Pesto

- Dinner: Roasted Vegetable Tacos
- Snack: Cottage Cheese with Pineapple
- Dessert: Peanut Butter and Banana Bites

Day 27

- Breakfast: Multigrain Muffins with Zucchini
- Lunch: Spinach and Strawberry Salad with Walnuts
- Dinner: Broccoli and Tofu Stir-Fry
- Snack: Almond Butter on Whole Grain Crackers
- Dessert: Roasted Pears with Honey

Day 28

- Breakfast: Breakfast Burrito with Avocado and Salsa
- Lunch: Edamame and Kale Salad
- Dinner: Chickpea and Spinach Curry
- Snack: Celery Sticks with Peanut Butter
- Dessert: Raw Date and Nut Bars

Day 29

- Breakfast: Chia Pudding with Coconut Milk and Mango
- Lunch: Roasted Beet and Goat Cheese Salad
- Dinner: Ratatouille with Brown Rice
- Snack: Mini Veggie Frittatas
- Dessert: Lemon Blueberry Muffins

Day 30

- Breakfast: Whole Wheat Bagel with Hummus and Cucumber
- Lunch: Vegan Sushi Rolls with Avocado and Cucumber
- Dinner: Vegan Shepherd's Pie
- Snack: Roasted Pumpkin Seeds
- Dessert: Apple Cinnamon Oatmeal Bars

Chapter 2: Breakfast Recipes

Breakfast is the most important meal of the day, especially for those managing pre-diabetes. A nutritious, balanced breakfast can help stabilize blood sugar levels and provide sustained energy throughout the morning. This chapter offers a variety of vegetarian breakfast recipes that are not only delicious but also packed with essential nutrients.

Avocado Toast with Tomatoes and Microgreens

Ingredients:

- 1 slice whole grain bread
- 1/2 ripe avocado
- 5 cherry tomatoes, halved
- Handful of microgreens
- Salt and pepper to taste
- 1 tsp olive oil

Instructions:

1. Toast the bread until golden brown.
2. Mash the avocado and spread it evenly over the toast.
3. Top with cherry tomatoes and microgreens.

4. Drizzle with olive oil and season with salt and pepper.

Nutrition Information:

- Calories: 250
- Protein: 4g
- Carbohydrates: 28g
- Fat: 15g
- Fiber: 8g
- Sugar: 3g
- Portion size: 1 toast

Quinoa Breakfast Bowl with Berries and Almonds

Ingredients:

- 1/2 cup cooked quinoa
- 1/4 cup mixed berries (blueberries, raspberries, strawberries)
- 1 tbsp sliced almonds
- 1 tbsp honey or maple syrup
- 1/4 cup unsweetened almond milk

Instructions:

1. Place cooked quinoa in a bowl.
2. Top with mixed berries and sliced almonds.

3. Drizzle with honey or maple syrup.

4. Pour almond milk over the top.

Nutrition Information:

- Calories: 300

- Protein: 8g

- Carbohydrates: 45g

- Fat: 9g

- Fiber: 6g

- Sugar: 15g

- Portion size: 1 bowl

Greek Yogurt with Chia Seeds and Fresh Fruit

Ingredients:

- 1 cup Greek yogurt

- 1 tbsp chia seeds

- 1/2 cup mixed fresh fruit (e.g., berries, banana, kiwi)

- 1 tsp honey (optional)

Instructions:

1. Mix chia seeds into the Greek yogurt.

2. Top with mixed fresh fruit.

3. Drizzle with honey if desired.

Nutrition Information:

- Calories: 220
- Protein: 15g
- Carbohydrates: 20g
- Fat: 8g
- Fiber: 5g
- Sugar: 15g
- Portion size: 1 cup

Spinach and Mushroom Frittata

Ingredients:

- 2 eggs
- 1/2 cup spinach, chopped
- 1/4 cup mushrooms, sliced
- 1 tbsp olive oil
- Salt and pepper to taste

Instructions:

1. Preheat oven to 375°F (190°C).
2. Sauté mushrooms in olive oil until soft.
3. Add spinach and cook until wilted.

4. Beat eggs and pour over the vegetables.

5. Cook on stovetop for 2 minutes, then transfer to the oven and bake for 10 minutes.

Nutrition Information:

- Calories: 200
- Protein: 12g
- Carbohydrates: 3g
- Fat: 15g
- Fiber: 2g
- Sugar: 1g
- Portion size: 1 frittata

Overnight Oats with Flaxseeds and Blueberries

Ingredients:

- 1/2 cup rolled oats
- 1 tbsp flaxseeds
- 1/2 cup blueberries
- 1 cup unsweetened almond milk
- 1 tsp honey or maple syrup

Instructions:

1. Combine oats, flaxseeds, and almond milk in a jar.

2. Stir in blueberries and honey.

3. Cover and refrigerate overnight.

Nutrition Information:

- Calories: 250

- Protein: 6g

- Carbohydrates: 40g

- Fat: 8g

- Fiber: 8g

- Sugar: 10g

- Portion size: 1 jar

Whole Grain Pancakes with Fresh Strawberries

Ingredients:

- 1 cup whole grain flour

- 1 tsp baking powder

- 1 egg

- 1 cup unsweetened almond milk

- 1 tbsp honey

- 1 cup fresh strawberries, sliced

Instructions:

1. Mix flour and baking powder in a bowl.
2. Beat the egg and add to the flour mixture along with almond milk and honey.
3. Stir until smooth.
4. Pour batter onto a hot griddle and cook until bubbles form, then flip.
5. Serve with fresh strawberries on top.

Nutrition Information:

- Calories: 300
- Protein: 10g
- Carbohydrates: 55g
- Fat: 6g
- Fiber: 8g
- Sugar: 12g
- Portion size: 2 pancakes

Smoothie Bowl with Nuts and Seeds

Ingredients:

- 1 banana, frozen
- 1/2 cup frozen berries
- 1/2 cup unsweetened almond milk

- 1 tbsp almond butter
- 1 tbsp chia seeds
- 1 tbsp pumpkin seeds
- 1/4 cup granola

Instructions:

1. Blend banana, berries, almond milk, and almond butter until smooth.
2. Pour into a bowl and top with chia seeds, pumpkin seeds, and granola.

Nutrition Information:

- Calories: 350
- Protein: 8g
- Carbohydrates: 55g
- Fat: 12g
- Fiber: 10g
- Sugar: 20g
- Portion size: 1 bowl

Scrambled Tofu with Veggies

Ingredients:

- 1/2 block firm tofu, crumbled

- 1/2 cup spinach, chopped
- 1/4 cup bell pepper, diced
- 1/4 cup onion, diced
- 1 tbsp olive oil
- 1/2 tsp turmeric
- Salt and pepper to taste

Instructions:

1. Heat olive oil in a pan.
2. Add onion and bell pepper, cook until soft.
3. Add crumbled tofu and turmeric, stir well.
4. Add spinach and cook until wilted.
5. Season with salt and pepper.

Nutrition Information:

- Calories: 200
- Protein: 15g
- Carbohydrates: 8g
- Fat: 12g
- Fiber: 4g
- Sugar: 3g
- Portion size: 1 serving

Sweet Potato Hash with Black Beans

Ingredients:

- 1 sweet potato, diced
- 1/2 cup black beans, rinsed and drained
- 1/4 cup onion, diced
- 1/4 cup bell pepper, diced
- 1 tbsp olive oil
- 1/2 tsp cumin
- Salt and pepper to taste

Instructions:

1. Heat olive oil in a skillet.
2. Add sweet potato, onion, and bell pepper, cook until soft.
3. Add black beans and cumin, stir well.
4. Season with salt and pepper.

Nutrition Information:

- Calories: 250
- Protein: 6g
- Carbohydrates: 45g
- Fat: 8g
- Fiber: 10g
- Sugar: 8g
- Portion size: 1 serving

Oatmeal with Apple Slices and Cinnamon

Ingredients:

- 1/2 cup rolled oats
- 1 cup water or unsweetened almond milk
- 1 apple, sliced
- 1/2 tsp cinnamon
- 1 tsp honey or maple syrup

Instructions:

1. Cook oats in water or almond milk according to package instructions.
2. Top with apple slices, cinnamon, and honey.

Nutrition Information:

- Calories: 220
- Protein: 5g
- Carbohydrates: 40g
- Fat: 4g
- Fiber: 6g
- Sugar: 15g
- Portion size: 1 bowl

Buckwheat Porridge with Banana and Walnuts

Ingredients:

- 1/2 cup buckwheat groats
- 1 cup water or unsweetened almond milk
- 1 banana, sliced
- 1 tbsp chopped walnuts
- 1 tsp honey or maple syrup

Instructions:

1. Cook buckwheat groats in water or almond milk according to package instructions.
2. Top with banana slices, walnuts, and honey.

Nutrition Information:

- Calories: 300
- Protein: 8g
- Carbohydrates: 55g
- Fat: 8g
- Fiber: 8g
- Sugar: 15g
- Portion size: 1 bowl

Multigrain Muffins with Zucchini

Ingredients:

- 1 cup whole wheat flour
- 1/2 cup rolled oats
- 1/2 cup grated zucchini
- 1/4 cup honey or maple syrup
- 1/4 cup unsweetened applesauce
- 1 tsp baking powder
- 1/2 tsp baking soda
- 1 tsp cinnamon

Instructions:

1. Preheat oven to 350°F (175°C).
2. Mix all ingredients in a bowl until well combined.
3. Spoon batter into a muffin tin.
4. Bake for 20-25 minutes or until a toothpick comes out clean.

Nutrition Information:

- Calories: 180
- Protein: 4g
- Carbohydrates: 30g
- Fat: 4g
- Fiber: 4g
- Sugar: 12g

- Portion size: 1 muffin

Breakfast Burrito with Avocado and Salsa

Ingredients:

- 1 whole wheat tortilla
- 1/2 avocado, sliced
- 1/4 cup black beans, rinsed and drained
- 1/4 cup salsa
- 1/4 cup shredded lettuce

Instructions:

1. Layer avocado, black beans, salsa, and lettuce on the tortilla.
2. Roll up and serve.

Nutrition Information:

- Calories: 300
- Protein: 8g
- Carbohydrates: 45g
- Fat: 12g
- Fiber: 12g
- Sugar: 4g
- Portion size: 1 burrito

Chia Pudding with Coconut Milk and Mango

Ingredients:

- 1/4 cup chia seeds
- 1 cup coconut milk
- 1 tbsp honey or maple syrup
- 1/2 cup diced mango

Instructions:

1. Mix chia seeds, coconut milk, and honey in a bowl.
2. Refrigerate for at least 2 hours or overnight.
3. Top with diced mango before serving.

Nutrition Information:

- Calories: 250
- Protein: 4g
- Carbohydrates: 30g
- Fat: 15g
- Fiber: 10g
- Sugar: 15g
- Portion size: 1 cup

Whole Wheat Bagel with Hummus and Cucumber

Ingredients:

- 1 whole wheat bagel
- 2 tbsp hummus
- 1/2 cucumber, sliced
- Salt and pepper to taste

Instructions:

1. Slice the bagel in half and toast.
2. Spread hummus on each half.
3. Top with cucumber slices.
4. Season with salt and pepper.

Nutrition Information:

- Calories: 250
- Protein: 8g
- Carbohydrates: 45g
- Fat: 6g
- Fiber: 8g
- Sugar: 5g
- Portion size: 1 bagel

Chapter 3: Lunch Recipes

Eating a balanced and nutritious lunch is crucial for managing prediabetes. The following recipes are designed to be both delicious and health-conscious, focusing on whole, plant-based ingredients that help maintain stable blood sugar levels. Each recipe is packed with nutrients, fiber, and healthy fats to keep you energized throughout the day.

Lentil Salad with Feta and Spinach

Ingredients:

- 1 cup cooked lentils
- 2 cups fresh spinach, chopped
- 1/2 cup crumbled feta cheese
- 1/2 cup cherry tomatoes, halved
- 1/4 cup red onion, finely chopped
- 2 tablespoons olive oil
- 1 tablespoon balsamic vinegar
- Salt and pepper to taste

Instructions:

1. In a large bowl, combine the lentils, spinach, feta cheese, cherry tomatoes, and red onion.

2. Drizzle with olive oil and balsamic vinegar.

3. Season with salt and pepper, and toss to combine.

Nutrition Information (per serving):

- Calories: 320
- Protein: 15g
- Carbohydrates: 28g
- Fat: 18g
- Fiber: 10g
- Sugar: 4g
- Portion size: 1 bowl

Chickpea and Avocado Sandwich

Ingredients:

- 1 can chickpeas, drained and mashed
- 1 avocado, mashed
- 1 tablespoon lemon juice
- 1/4 cup red onion, chopped
- 2 tablespoons fresh cilantro, chopped
- Salt and pepper to taste
- 4 slices whole grain bread
- Lettuce leaves

Instructions:

1. In a bowl, mix the mashed chickpeas, avocado, lemon juice, red onion, cilantro, salt, and pepper.
2. Spread the mixture onto two slices of whole grain bread.
3. Top with lettuce leaves and the remaining bread slices.

Nutrition Information (per serving):

- Calories: 350
- Protein: 12g
- Carbohydrates: 42g
- Fat: 15g
- Fiber: 14g
- Sugar: 5g
- Portion size: 1 sandwich

Quinoa Salad with Roasted Vegetables

Ingredients:

- 1 cup quinoa, cooked
- 1 cup roasted vegetables (bell peppers, zucchini, eggplant)
- 1/4 cup feta cheese, crumbled
- 2 tablespoons olive oil
- 1 tablespoon lemon juice
- Salt and pepper to taste

Instructions:

1. In a large bowl, combine the cooked quinoa, roasted vegetables, and feta cheese.
2. Drizzle with olive oil and lemon juice.
3. Season with salt and pepper, and toss to combine.

Nutrition Information (per serving):

- Calories: 280
- Protein: 9g
- Carbohydrates: 34g
- Fat: 12g
- Fiber: 6g
- Sugar: 4g
- Portion size: 1 bowl

Vegetable Stir-Fry with Tofu

Ingredients:

- 1 block tofu, cubed
- 2 cups mixed vegetables (broccoli, bell peppers, carrots)
- 2 tablespoons soy sauce
- 1 tablespoon sesame oil
- 1 clove garlic, minced
- 1 teaspoon ginger, grated

Instructions:

1. In a pan, heat sesame oil and sauté garlic and ginger until fragrant.
2. Add tofu cubes and stir-fry until golden brown.
3. Add mixed vegetables and soy sauce, and cook until vegetables are tender.

Nutrition Information (per serving):

- Calories: 250
- Protein: 15g
- Carbohydrates: 12g
- Fat: 16g
- Fiber: 5g
- Sugar: 3g
- Portion size: 1 bowl

Caprese Salad with Balsamic Glaze

Ingredients:

- 2 cups cherry tomatoes, halved
- 1 cup fresh mozzarella balls, halved
- 1/4 cup fresh basil leaves
- 2 tablespoons balsamic glaze
- 1 tablespoon olive oil

- Salt and pepper to taste

Instructions:

1. In a bowl, combine cherry tomatoes, mozzarella, and basil leaves.
2. Drizzle with balsamic glaze and olive oil.
3. Season with salt and pepper, and toss to combine.

Nutrition Information (per serving):

- Calories: 200
- Protein: 10g
- Carbohydrates: 12g
- Fat: 14g
- Fiber: 2g
- Sugar: 6g
- Portion size: 1 bowl

Mediterranean Chickpea Bowl

Ingredients:

- 1 cup cooked chickpeas
- 1/2 cup cucumber, diced
- 1/2 cup cherry tomatoes, halved
- 1/4 cup red onion, finely chopped

- 1/4 cup kalamata olives, pitted and sliced
- 2 tablespoons feta cheese, crumbled
- 2 tablespoons olive oil
- 1 tablespoon lemon juice
- Salt and pepper to taste

Instructions:

1. In a bowl, combine chickpeas, cucumber, cherry tomatoes, red onion, olives, and feta cheese.
2. Drizzle with olive oil and lemon juice.
3. Season with salt and pepper, and toss to combine.

Nutrition Information (per serving):

- Calories: 300
- Protein: 10g
- Carbohydrates: 28g
- Fat: 18g
- Fiber: 8g
- Sugar: 5g
- Portion size: 1 bowl

Black Bean and Corn Salad

Ingredients:

- 1 can black beans, drained and rinsed
- 1 cup corn kernels
- 1/2 cup red bell pepper, diced
- 1/4 cup red onion, finely chopped
- 1/4 cup fresh cilantro, chopped
- 2 tablespoons olive oil
- 1 tablespoon lime juice
- Salt and pepper to taste

Instructions:

1. In a bowl, combine black beans, corn, red bell pepper, red onion, and cilantro.
2. Drizzle with olive oil and lime juice.
3. Season with salt and pepper, and toss to combine.

Nutrition Information (per serving):

- Calories: 220
- Protein: 8g
- Carbohydrates: 36g
- Fat: 6g
- Fiber: 10g
- Sugar: 4g

- Portion size: 1 bowl

Veggie Wrap with Hummus and Sprouts

Ingredients:

- 1 whole wheat tortilla
- 1/4 cup hummus
- 1/2 cup mixed vegetables (carrots, bell peppers, cucumber), julienned
- 1/4 cup alfalfa sprouts
- 1 tablespoon sunflower seeds

Instructions:

1. Spread hummus over the tortilla.
2. Add mixed vegetables and alfalfa sprouts.
3. Sprinkle with sunflower seeds, roll up the tortilla, and slice in half.

Nutrition Information (per serving):

- Calories: 250
- Protein: 8g
- Carbohydrates: 35g
- Fat: 10g
- Fiber: 8g

- Sugar: 3g
- Portion size: 1 wrap

Greek Salad with Olives and Cucumber

Ingredients:

- 2 cups romaine lettuce, chopped
- 1/2 cup cherry tomatoes, halved
- 1/2 cup cucumber, sliced
- 1/4 cup red onion, thinly sliced
- 1/4 cup kalamata olives, pitted and sliced
- 1/4 cup feta cheese, crumbled
- 2 tablespoons olive oil
- 1 tablespoon red wine vinegar
- Salt and pepper to taste

Instructions:

1. In a bowl, combine romaine lettuce, cherry tomatoes, cucumber, red onion, olives, and feta cheese.
2. Drizzle with olive oil and red wine vinegar.
3. Season with salt and pepper, and toss to combine.

Nutrition Information (per serving):

- Calories: 210

- Protein: 6g

- Carbohydrates: 12g

- Fat: 16g

- Fiber: 4g

- Sugar: 5g

- Portion size: 1 bowl

Sweet Potato and Black Bean Tacos

Ingredients:

- 2 sweet potatoes, peeled and diced

- 1 can black beans, drained and rinsed

- 1/2 cup red bell pepper, diced

- 1/4 cup red onion, chopped

- 1 tablespoon olive oil

- 1 teaspoon cumin

- Salt and pepper to taste

- 4 small corn tortillas

- Fresh cilantro for garnish

Instructions:

1. Preheat oven to 400°F (200°C). Toss sweet potatoes with olive oil, cumin, salt, and pepper. Roast for 20 minutes.

2. In a bowl, combine roasted sweet potatoes, black beans, red bell pepper, and red onion.
3. Warm the tortillas and fill with the sweet potato mixture.
4. Garnish with fresh cilantro.

Nutrition Information (per serving):

- Calories: 280
- Protein: 8g
- Carbohydrates: 52g
- Fat: 5g
- Fiber: 12g
- Sugar: 8g
- Portion size: 2 tacos

Cauliflower Rice with Pesto

Ingredients:

- 1 head cauliflower, riced
- 1/4 cup basil pesto
- 1/2 cup cherry tomatoes, halved
- 1/4 cup pine nuts, toasted
- 1 tablespoon olive oil
- Salt and pepper to taste

Instructions:

1. Heat olive oil in a pan and sauté the cauliflower rice until tender, about 5 minutes.
2. Stir in the pesto and cherry tomatoes.
3. Top with toasted pine nuts and season with salt and pepper.

Nutrition Information (per serving):

- Calories: 220
- Protein: 6g
- Carbohydrates: 16g
- Fat: 16g
- Fiber: 6g
- Sugar: 5g
- Portion size: 1 bowl

Spinach and Strawberry Salad with Walnuts

Ingredients:

- 2 cups fresh spinach
- 1 cup strawberries, sliced
- 1/4 cup walnuts, chopped
- 2 tablespoons feta cheese, crumbled
- 2 tablespoons balsamic vinaigrette

Instructions:

1. In a bowl, combine spinach, strawberries, walnuts, and feta cheese.

2. Drizzle with balsamic vinaigrette and toss to combine.

Nutrition Information (per serving):

- Calories: 190
- Protein: 5g
- Carbohydrates: 15g
- Fat: 14g
- Fiber: 4g
- Sugar: 8g
- Portion size: 1 bowl

Edamame and Kale Salad

Ingredients:

- 2 cups kale, chopped
- 1 cup shelled edamame, cooked
- 1/4 cup red bell pepper, diced
- 1/4 cup carrot, grated
- 2 tablespoons sesame seeds
- 2 tablespoons soy sauce
- 1 tablespoon rice vinegar

- 1 teaspoon sesame oil

Instructions:

1. In a bowl, combine kale, edamame, red bell pepper, carrot, and sesame seeds.
2. Drizzle with soy sauce, rice vinegar, and sesame oil.
3. Toss to combine.

Nutrition Information (per serving):

- Calories: 180
- Protein: 10g
- Carbohydrates: 18g
- Fat: 8g
- Fiber: 6g
- Sugar: 4g
- Portion size: 1 bowl

Roasted Beet and Goat Cheese Salad

Ingredients:

- 2 beets, roasted and sliced
- 2 cups mixed greens
- 1/4 cup goat cheese, crumbled
- 1/4 cup walnuts, toasted

- 2 tablespoons balsamic vinaigrette

Instructions:

1. In a bowl, combine roasted beets, mixed greens, goat cheese, and walnuts.
2. Drizzle with balsamic vinaigrette and toss to combine.

Nutrition Information (per serving):

- Calories: 230
- Protein: 7g
- Carbohydrates: 17g
- Fat: 16g
- Fiber: 5g
- Sugar: 9g
- Portion size: 1 bowl

Vegan Sushi Rolls with Avocado and Cucumber

Ingredients:

- 1 cup sushi rice, cooked
- 1 tablespoon rice vinegar
- 4 nori sheets
- 1 avocado, sliced

- 1/2 cucumber, julienned
- 1/4 cup carrot, julienned
- Soy sauce for dipping

Instructions:

1. Mix cooked sushi rice with rice vinegar.
2. Place a nori sheet on a bamboo mat, spread a thin layer of rice over it.
3. Add avocado, cucumber, and carrot.
4. Roll tightly and slice into pieces. Serve with soy sauce.

Nutrition Information (per serving):

- Calories: 200
- Protein: 4g
- Carbohydrates: 38g
- Fat: 6g
- Fiber: 6g
- Sugar: 2g
- Portion size: 1 roll

Chapter 4: Dinner Recipes

In this chapter, you'll find a variety of nutritious and delicious dinner recipes designed for those following a vegetarian diet, especially beneficial for managing pre-diabetes. Each recipe focuses on wholesome ingredients and simple preparations to help you maintain a balanced approach to eating. From stuffed peppers to hearty stews and flavorful pasta dishes, these recipes aim to satisfy both your taste buds and nutritional needs.

Stuffed Bell Peppers with Quinoa and Vegetables

Ingredients:

- 4 large bell peppers, any color
- 1 cup quinoa, rinsed
- 2 cups vegetable broth
- 1 onion, diced
- 2 cloves garlic, minced
- 1 zucchini, diced
- 1 cup cherry tomatoes, halved
- 1 teaspoon dried oregano
- Salt and pepper, to taste
- Fresh parsley, for garnish

Instructions:

1. Preheat oven to 375°F (190°C). Cut the tops off the bell peppers and remove seeds.
2. In a saucepan, bring vegetable broth to a boil. Add quinoa, reduce heat, cover, and simmer for 15 minutes or until quinoa is cooked.
3. In a separate pan, sauté onion and garlic until softened. Add zucchini, cherry tomatoes, oregano, salt, and pepper. Cook until vegetables are tender.
4. Stir cooked quinoa into the vegetable mixture. Spoon mixture into bell peppers.
5. Place stuffed peppers in a baking dish. Cover with foil and bake for 25-30 minutes, until peppers are tender.
6. Garnish with fresh parsley before serving.

Nutrition Information (per serving):

- Calories: 280
- Protein: 9g
- Carbohydrates: 53g
- Fat: 4g
- Fiber: 9g
- Sugar: 8g
- Portion size: 1 stuffed pepper

Eggplant Parmesan with Whole Wheat Pasta

Ingredients:

- 1 large eggplant, sliced into rounds
- 1 cup whole wheat breadcrumbs
- 1 cup grated Parmesan cheese
- 2 cups marinara sauce
- 8 oz whole wheat pasta
- Fresh basil leaves, for garnish

Instructions:

1. Preheat oven to 400°F (200°C). Line a baking sheet with parchment paper.
2. Dip eggplant slices in beaten egg, then coat with breadcrumbs mixed with Parmesan cheese.
3. Arrange coated eggplant slices on the baking sheet. Bake for 20 minutes, flipping halfway through, until golden brown.
4. Cook pasta according to package instructions. Drain and set aside.
5. In a saucepan, heat marinara sauce until warmed through.
6. To serve, place a portion of pasta on each plate, top with marinara sauce, and arrange baked eggplant slices on top. Garnish with fresh basil.

Nutrition Information (per serving):

- Calories: 420
- Protein: 18g
- Carbohydrates: 68g
- Fat: 9g
- Fiber: 12g
- Sugar: 12g
- Portion size: 1/4 of recipe

Veggie Burger with Sweet Potato Fries

Ingredients:

- 4 veggie burger patties (store-bought or homemade)
- 4 whole wheat burger buns
- Lettuce leaves, tomato slices, onion slices (for topping)
- 2 large sweet potatoes, peeled and cut into fries
- 2 tablespoons olive oil
- 1 teaspoon paprika
- Salt and pepper, to taste

Instructions:

1. Preheat oven to 425°F (220°C). Line a baking sheet with parchment paper.

2. Toss sweet potato fries with olive oil, paprika, salt, and pepper until evenly coated. Spread in a single layer on the baking sheet.

3. Bake fries for 25-30 minutes, flipping halfway through, until crispy and golden brown.

4. While fries are baking, cook veggie burger patties according to package instructions or homemade recipe.

5. Toast burger buns if desired. Assemble burgers with lettuce, tomato, onion, and veggie patties.

6. Serve burgers with a side of sweet potato fries.

Nutrition Information (per serving, including fries):

- Calories: 450
- Protein: 15g
- Carbohydrates: 70g
- Fat: 13g
- Fiber: 12g
- Sugar: 12g
- Portion size: 1 burger with fries

Spaghetti Squash with Marinara Sauce

Ingredients:

- 1 medium spaghetti squash

- 2 cups marinara sauce (store-bought or homemade)
- Fresh basil leaves, for garnish
- Grated Parmesan cheese (optional)

Instructions:

1. Preheat oven to 400°F (200°C). Cut spaghetti squash in half lengthwise and scoop out seeds.
2. Place squash halves cut-side down on a baking sheet lined with parchment paper. Bake for 40-50 minutes until tender.
3. Let squash cool slightly, then use a fork to scrape out the strands into a bowl.
4. Heat marinara sauce in a saucepan until warmed through.
5. Serve spaghetti squash topped with marinara sauce. Garnish with fresh basil and Parmesan cheese if desired.

Nutrition Information (per serving):
- Calories: 220
- Protein: 5g
- Carbohydrates: 40g
- Fat: 6g
- Fiber: 8g
- Sugar: 12g
- Portion size: 1/2 squash with sauce

Lentil and Vegetable Stew

Ingredients:

- 1 cup green lentils, rinsed
- 4 cups vegetable broth
- 1 onion, diced
- 2 carrots, diced
- 2 celery stalks, diced
- 2 cloves garlic, minced
- 1 teaspoon dried thyme
- 1 teaspoon paprika
- Salt and pepper, to taste
- Fresh parsley, for garnish

Instructions:

1. In a large pot, combine lentils and vegetable broth. Bring to a boil, then reduce heat and simmer for 20 minutes.
2. In a separate pan, sauté onion, carrots, celery, and garlic until softened.
3. Add sautéed vegetables to the pot with lentils. Stir in dried thyme, paprika, salt, and pepper.
4. Simmer stew for an additional 10-15 minutes until flavors are combined and vegetables are tender.
5. Serve hot, garnished with fresh parsley.

Nutrition Information (per serving):

- Calories: 280
- Protein: 18g
- Carbohydrates: 50g
- Fat: 1g
- Fiber: 18g
- Sugar: 5g
- Portion size: 1/4 of recipe

Cauliflower Pizza with Fresh Tomatoes and Basil

Ingredients:

- 1 cauliflower pizza crust (store-bought or homemade)
- 1 cup marinara sauce
- 1 cup cherry tomatoes, halved
- 1 cup shredded mozzarella cheese (or vegan cheese)
- Fresh basil leaves, for garnish

Instructions:

1. Preheat oven according to crust package instructions or homemade recipe.
2. Spread marinara sauce evenly over cauliflower crust.
3. Top with cherry tomatoes and shredded mozzarella cheese.

4. Bake pizza according to crust package instructions, until cheese is melted and crust is golden brown.

5. Remove from oven and garnish with fresh basil leaves before serving.

Nutrition Information (per serving):

- Calories: 300
- Protein: 15g
- Carbohydrates: 30g
- Fat: 15g
- Fiber: 8g
- Sugar: 8g
- Portion size: 1/4 of pizza

Zucchini Noodles with Avocado Pesto

Ingredients:

- 4 medium zucchinis, spiralized into noodles
- 1 avocado, peeled and pitted
- 1 cup fresh basil leaves
- 1 clove garlic, minced
- 1/4 cup pine nuts
- 2 tablespoons lemon juice
- 3 tablespoons olive oil

- Salt and pepper, to taste
- Cherry tomatoes, halved, for garnish

Instructions:

1. In a blender or food processor, combine avocado, basil, garlic, pine nuts, lemon juice, olive oil, salt, and pepper. Blend until smooth and creamy.
2. In a large pan, heat a tablespoon of olive oil over medium heat. Add zucchini noodles and sauté for 2-3 minutes until tender but still crisp.
3. Remove noodles from heat and toss with avocado pesto until well coated.
4. Serve immediately, garnished with cherry tomatoes.

Nutrition Information (per serving):

- Calories: 250
- Protein: 6g
- Carbohydrates: 15g
- Fat: 20g
- Fiber: 8g
- Sugar: 6g
- Portion size: 1/4 of recipe

Baked Falafel with Tzatziki

Ingredients:

- 2 cups cooked chickpeas, drained and rinsed
- 1/2 onion, chopped
- 2 cloves garlic, minced
- 1/4 cup fresh parsley
- 1 teaspoon ground cumin
- 1 teaspoon ground coriander
- 1/2 teaspoon baking powder
- Salt and pepper, to taste
- Olive oil cooking spray
- Tzatziki sauce (store-bought or homemade), for serving

Instructions:

1. Preheat oven to 375°F (190°C). Line a baking sheet with parchment paper and spray with olive oil cooking spray.
2. In a food processor, combine chickpeas, onion, garlic, parsley, cumin, coriander, baking powder, salt, and pepper. Pulse until mixture is well combined and forms a coarse paste.
3. Form mixture into golf ball-sized balls and place on the prepared baking sheet. Flatten slightly with the back of a spoon.

4. Spray the tops of the falafel with olive oil cooking spray. Bake for 20-25 minutes, flipping halfway through, until falafel are golden brown and crispy.

5. Serve hot with tzatziki sauce for dipping.

Nutrition Information (per serving, without tzatziki):

- Calories: 180
- Protein: 8g
- Carbohydrates: 28g
- Fat: 4g
- Fiber: 6g
- Sugar: 5g
- Portion size: 4 falafel

Spinach and Ricotta Stuffed Shells

Ingredients:

- 20 jumbo pasta shells
- 2 cups ricotta cheese (or tofu ricotta for vegan option)
- 1 cup chopped spinach, cooked and drained
- 1/2 cup grated Parmesan cheese (or nutritional yeast for vegan option)
- 1 egg (or flaxseed egg for vegan option)
- 1 teaspoon dried oregano

- Salt and pepper, to taste
- 2 cups marinara sauce
- Fresh basil leaves, for garnish

Instructions:

1. Cook pasta shells according to package instructions until al dente. Drain and set aside.
2. Preheat oven to 375°F (190°C). Grease a baking dish with olive oil or cooking spray.
3. In a bowl, combine ricotta cheese (or tofu ricotta), spinach, Parmesan cheese (or nutritional yeast), egg (or flaxseed egg), oregano, salt, and pepper.
4. Stuff each cooked pasta shell with the ricotta mixture and place in the prepared baking dish.
5. Pour marinara sauce over the stuffed shells. Cover with foil and bake for 25-30 minutes, until heated through.
6. Garnish with fresh basil leaves before serving.

Nutrition Information (per serving):

- Calories: 350
- Protein: 20g
- Carbohydrates: 45g
- Fat: 10g
- Fiber: 5g

- Sugar: 8g
- Portion size: 5 shells

Mushroom and Spinach Risotto

Ingredients:

- 1 cup Arborio rice
- 4 cups vegetable broth
- 1 tablespoon olive oil
- 1 onion, diced
- 2 cloves garlic, minced
- 8 oz mushrooms, sliced
- 2 cups baby spinach
- 1/2 cup grated Parmesan cheese (or nutritional yeast for vegan option)
- Salt and pepper, to taste
- Fresh parsley, for garnish

Instructions:

1. In a saucepan, bring vegetable broth to a simmer and keep warm.
2. In a large pan, heat olive oil over medium heat. Add onion and garlic, sauté until softened.

3. Add mushrooms to the pan and cook until they release their juices and are browned.

4. Stir in Arborio rice and cook for 1-2 minutes until rice is translucent around the edges.

5. Gradually add warm vegetable broth, 1/2 cup at a time, stirring constantly and allowing each addition to be absorbed before adding more.

6. Continue adding broth and stirring until rice is creamy and cooked al dente, about 20-25 minutes.

7. Stir in baby spinach and Parmesan cheese (or nutritional yeast). Season with salt and pepper.

8. Remove from heat and let rest for a few minutes before serving.

9. Garnish with fresh parsley before serving.

Nutrition Information (per serving):

- Calories: 400
- Protein: 12g
- Carbohydrates: 60g
- Fat: 12g
- Fiber: 5g
- Sugar: 3g
- Portion size: 1/4 of recipe

Roasted Vegetable Tacos

Ingredients:

- 1 large sweet potato, peeled and cubed
- 1 red bell pepper, sliced
- 1 yellow bell pepper, sliced
- 1 red onion, sliced
- 1 tablespoon olive oil
- 1 teaspoon chili powder
- 1/2 teaspoon cumin
- Salt and pepper, to taste
- 8 small corn or flour tortillas
- 1 cup black beans, cooked and drained
- Fresh cilantro, for garnish
- Lime wedges, for serving

Instructions:

1. Preheat oven to 400°F (200°C). Line a baking sheet with parchment paper.
2. In a bowl, toss sweet potato, bell peppers, and red onion with olive oil, chili powder, cumin, salt, and pepper until evenly coated.
3. Spread vegetables in a single layer on the prepared baking sheet. Roast for 20-25 minutes, stirring halfway through, until vegetables are tender and lightly browned.

4. Heat tortillas according to package instructions or preference.

5. To assemble tacos, spread a spoonful of black beans on each tortilla. Top with roasted vegetables.

6. Garnish with fresh cilantro and serve with lime wedges for squeezing over tacos.

Nutrition Information (per serving, 2 tacos):

- Calories: 320
- Protein: 10g
- Carbohydrates: 55g
- Fat: 8g
- Fiber: 10g
- Sugar: 8g
- Portion size: 2 tacos

Broccoli and Tofu Stir-Fry

Ingredients:

- 1 block firm tofu, pressed and cubed
- 2 tablespoons soy sauce
- 1 tablespoon sesame oil
- 1 tablespoon cornstarch
- 1 tablespoon olive oil

- 2 cups broccoli florets

- 1 red bell pepper, sliced

- 1 carrot, sliced into matchsticks

- 2 cloves garlic, minced

- 1 tablespoon grated ginger

- Cooked brown rice, for serving

Instructions:

1. In a bowl, toss cubed tofu with soy sauce, sesame oil, and cornstarch until tofu is coated.

2. Heat olive oil in a large pan or wok over medium-high heat. Add tofu and cook until golden and crispy on all sides. Remove tofu from pan and set aside.

3. In the same pan, add broccoli, bell pepper, carrot, garlic, and ginger. Stir-fry for 5-7 minutes until vegetables are tender-crisp.

4. Return tofu to the pan and stir to combine with vegetables.

5. Serve stir-fry over cooked brown rice.

Nutrition Information (per serving):

- Calories: 380

- Protein: 20g

- Carbohydrates: 35g

- Fat: 18g

* Fiber: 8g

* Sugar: 6g

* Portion size: 1/4 of recipe

Chickpea and Spinach Curry

Ingredients:

* 1 tablespoon olive oil

* 1 onion, finely chopped

* 2 cloves garlic, minced

* 1 tablespoon grated ginger

* 1 teaspoon ground cumin

* 1 teaspoon ground coriander

* 1/2 teaspoon turmeric powder

* 1/2 teaspoon paprika

* 1/4 teaspoon cayenne pepper (optional)

* 1 can (15 oz) chickpeas, drained and rinsed

* 1 can (14 oz) diced tomatoes

* 1 cup coconut milk

* 2 cups baby spinach

* Salt and pepper, to taste

* Fresh cilantro, for garnish

* Cooked brown rice or naan bread, for serving

Instructions:

1. Heat olive oil in a large skillet over medium heat. Add onion and sauté until softened.

2. Add garlic, ginger, cumin, coriander, turmeric, paprika, and cayenne pepper (if using). Cook for 1-2 minutes until fragrant.

3. Stir in chickpeas and diced tomatoes (with their juices). Simmer for 10 minutes, stirring occasionally.

4. Pour in coconut milk and bring to a simmer. Cook for another 5 minutes.

5. Add baby spinach and cook until wilted.

6. Season with salt and pepper to taste.

7. Serve hot over cooked brown rice or with naan bread, garnished with fresh cilantro.

Nutrition Information (per serving, without rice or naan):

- Calories: 320
- Protein: 12g
- Carbohydrates: 30g
- Fat: 18g
- Fiber: 8g
- Sugar: 7g
- Portion size: 1/4 of recipe

Ratatouille with Brown Rice

Ingredients:

- 1 eggplant, diced
- 2 zucchinis, diced
- 1 yellow bell pepper, diced
- 1 red bell pepper, diced
- 1 onion, diced
- 4 cloves garlic, minced
- 1 can (14 oz) diced tomatoes
- 2 tablespoons tomato paste
- 1 teaspoon dried thyme
- 1 teaspoon dried oregano
- Salt and pepper, to taste
- Fresh basil leaves, for garnish
- Cooked brown rice, for serving

Instructions:

1. Heat olive oil in a large pot or Dutch oven over medium heat. Add onion and garlic, sauté until softened.
2. Add eggplant, zucchinis, and bell peppers. Cook for 5-7 minutes until vegetables begin to soften.
3. Stir in diced tomatoes, tomato paste, thyme, oregano, salt, and pepper.

4. Bring to a simmer, then reduce heat to low. Cover and cook for 20-25 minutes, stirring occasionally, until vegetables are tender.

5. Serve hot over cooked brown rice, garnished with fresh basil.

Nutrition Information (per serving):

- Calories: 280
- Protein: 6g
- Carbohydrates: 50g
- Fat: 8g
- Fiber: 12g
- Sugar: 14g
- Portion size: 1/4 of recipe

Vegan Shepherd's Pie

Ingredients:

- 4 large potatoes, peeled and cubed
- 1 tablespoon olive oil
- 1 onion, diced
- 2 carrots, diced
- 2 celery stalks, diced
- 1 cup mushrooms, chopped

- 1 can (15 oz) lentils, drained and rinsed

- 1 cup frozen peas

- 2 tablespoons tomato paste

- 1 cup vegetable broth

- 1 teaspoon dried thyme

- Salt and pepper, to taste

- Fresh parsley, for garnish

Instructions:

1. Preheat oven to 375°F (190°C).

2. Boil potatoes in a large pot of water until tender, about 15 minutes. Drain and mash with a potato masher or fork. Season with salt and pepper.

3. In a large skillet, heat olive oil over medium heat. Add onion, carrots, and celery. Sauté until softened, about 5 minutes.

4. Add mushrooms to the skillet and cook until they release their juices and start to brown.

5. Stir in lentils, frozen peas, tomato paste, vegetable broth, thyme, salt, and pepper. Cook for 5-7 minutes until heated through and slightly thickened.

6. Transfer lentil mixture to a baking dish. Spread mashed potatoes evenly over the top.

7. Bake for 25-30 minutes, until the top is golden brown and the filling is bubbling.

8. Garnish with fresh parsley before serving.

Nutrition Information (per serving):

- Calories: 320
- Protein: 12g
- Carbohydrates: 60g
- Fat: 5g
- Fiber: 12g
- Sugar: 8g
- Portion size: 1/4 of recipe

Chapter 5: Snacks and Appetizers

In between meals, having healthy snacks can help maintain energy levels and prevent overeating later in the day. Here are delicious and nutritious snack and appetizer ideas that are perfect for anyone following a vegetarian diet.

Hummus with Carrot and Cucumber Sticks

Ingredients:

- Hummus
- Carrot sticks
- Cucumber sticks

Instructions:

1. Slice carrots and cucumbers into sticks.
2. Serve with a side of hummus for dipping.

Nutrition Information (per serving):

- Calories: 120
- Protein: 4g
- Carbohydrates: 15g
- Fat: 6g

- Fiber: 6g

- Sugar: 3g

- Portion size: 1/2 cup hummus with 1 cup vegetables

Baked Kale Chips

Ingredients:

- Fresh kale leaves

- Olive oil

- Salt

Instructions:

1. Preheat oven to 350°F (175°C).

2. Remove stems from kale leaves and tear into bite-sized pieces.

3. Toss with olive oil and spread on a baking sheet.

4. Sprinkle with salt.

5. Bake for 10-15 minutes until crispy.

Nutrition Information (per serving):

- Calories: 50

- Protein: 2g

- Carbohydrates: 6g

- Fat: 3g

- Fiber: 2g
- Sugar: 1g
- Portion size: 1 cup

Edamame with Sea Salt

Ingredients:

- Edamame (fresh or frozen)
- Sea salt

Instructions:

1. Steam or boil edamame according to package instructions.
2. Drain and sprinkle with sea salt.

Nutrition Information (per serving):

- Calories: 100
- Protein: 9g
- Carbohydrates: 9g
- Fat: 4g
- Fiber: 4g
- Sugar: 3g
- Portion size: 1 cup

Stuffed Mini Peppers with Goat Cheese

Ingredients:

- Mini bell peppers
- Goat cheese

Instructions:

1. Slice mini peppers in half lengthwise and remove seeds.
2. Fill each half with goat cheese.

Nutrition Information (per serving):

- Calories: 80
- Protein: 4g
- Carbohydrates: 5g
- Fat: 5g
- Fiber: 2g
- Sugar: 3g
- Portion size: 3 peppers

Avocado and Black Bean Salsa

Ingredients:

- Avocado
- Black beans
- Tomato

- Red onion
- Lime juice
- Cilantro
- Salt

Instructions:

1. Dice avocado, tomato, and red onion.
2. Mix with black beans, lime juice, cilantro, and salt.

Nutrition Information (per serving):

- Calories: 150
- Protein: 6g
- Carbohydrates: 20g
- Fat: 7g
- Fiber: 8g
- Sugar: 2g
- Portion size: 1/2 cup

Greek Yogurt with Fresh Fruit and Nuts

Ingredients:

- Greek yogurt
- Fresh fruit (e.g., berries, banana)
- Nuts (e.g., almonds, walnuts)

Instructions:

1. Spoon Greek yogurt into a bowl.
2. Top with fresh fruit and nuts.

Nutrition Information (per serving):

- Calories: 180
- Protein: 15g
- Carbohydrates: 15g
- Fat: 8g
- Fiber: 3g
- Sugar: 8g
- Portion size: 1 cup yogurt with 1/2 cup fruit and nuts

Spicy Roasted Chickpeas

Ingredients:

- Chickpeas (canned or cooked)
- Olive oil
- Paprika
- Cayenne pepper
- Salt

Instructions:

1. Preheat oven to 400°F (200°C).

2. Rinse and dry chickpeas.

3. Toss with olive oil, paprika, cayenne pepper, and salt.

4. Spread on a baking sheet and roast for 20-30 minutes until crispy.

Nutrition Information (per serving):

- Calories: 130

- Protein: 6g

- Carbohydrates: 18g

- Fat: 4g

- Fiber: 5g

- Sugar: 3g

- Portion size: 1/2 cup

Veggie Spring Rolls with Peanut Sauce

Ingredients:

- Rice paper wrappers

- Mixed vegetables (e.g., carrots, cucumber, lettuce)

- Fresh herbs (e.g., mint, cilantro)

- Peanut sauce

Instructions:

1. Dip rice paper wrappers in warm water to soften.

2. Fill with vegetables and herbs.

3. Roll tightly and serve with peanut sauce for dipping.

Nutrition Information (per serving):

- Calories: 120

- Protein: 3g

- Carbohydrates: 20g

- Fat: 3g

- Fiber: 4g

- Sugar: 3g

- Portion size: 2 rolls with 2 tbsp sauce

Caprese Skewers

Ingredients:

- Cherry tomatoes

- Fresh mozzarella balls (bocconcini)

- Fresh basil leaves

- Balsamic glaze

Instructions:

1. Thread cherry tomatoes, mozzarella balls, and basil leaves onto skewers.

2. Drizzle with balsamic glaze before serving.

Nutrition Information (per serving):

- Calories: 100
- Protein: 5g
- Carbohydrates: 5g
- Fat: 7g
- Fiber: 1g
- Sugar: 3g
- Portion size: 2 skewers

Guacamole with Whole Grain Tortilla Chips

Ingredients:

- Ripe avocados
- Tomato
- Red onion
- Lime juice
- Garlic
- Salt
- Whole grain tortilla chips

Instructions:

1. Mash avocados in a bowl.
2. Dice tomato and red onion; add to avocado.

3. Mix in lime juice, minced garlic, and salt to taste.

4. Serve with whole grain tortilla chips.

Nutrition Information (per serving):

- Calories: 160

- Protein: 3g

- Carbohydrates: 18g

- Fat: 9g

- Fiber: 7g

- Sugar: 2g

- Portion size: 1/2 cup guacamole with 10 chips

Cottage Cheese with Pineapple

Ingredients:

- Cottage cheese
- Fresh pineapple chunks

Instructions:

1. Spoon cottage cheese into a bowl.

2. Top with fresh pineapple chunks.

Nutrition Information (per serving):

- Calories: 120

- Protein: 15g

- Carbohydrates: 15g

- Fat: 2g

- Fiber: 2g

- Sugar: 12g

- Portion size: 1 cup

Almond Butter on Whole Grain Crackers

Ingredients:

- Whole grain crackers

- Almond butter

Instructions:

1. Spread almond butter on whole grain crackers.

Nutrition Information (per serving):

- Calories: 150

- Protein: 5g

- Carbohydrates: 20g

- Fat: 7g

- Fiber: 4g

- Sugar: 2g

- Portion size: 6 crackers with 2 tbsp almond butter

Celery Sticks with Peanut Butter

Ingredients:

- Celery sticks
- Peanut butter

Instructions:

1. Fill celery sticks with peanut butter.

Nutrition Information (per serving):

- Calories: 120
- Protein: 4g
- Carbohydrates: 8g
- Fat: 9g
- Fiber: 3g
- Sugar: 3g
- Portion size: 2 celery sticks with 2 tbsp peanut butter

Mini Veggie Frittatas

Ingredients:

- Eggs
- Mixed vegetables (e.g., spinach, bell peppers, tomatoes)
- Milk (or milk alternative)
- Cheese (optional)

- Salt and pepper

Instructions:

1. Preheat oven to 350°F (175°C).
2. Whisk eggs and milk together; season with salt and pepper.
3. Divide mixed vegetables and cheese (if using) into muffin tin cups.
4. Pour egg mixture over vegetables.
5. Bake for 20-25 minutes until set.

Nutrition Information (per serving):

- Calories: 100
- Protein: 8g
- Carbohydrates: 5g
- Fat: 5g
- Fiber: 1g
- Sugar: 2g
- Portion size: 2 mini frittatas

Roasted Pumpkin Seeds

Ingredients:

- Pumpkin seeds (raw)
- Olive oil

- Salt

Instructions:

1. Preheat oven to 300°F (150°C).

2. Toss pumpkin seeds with olive oil and salt.

3. Spread on a baking sheet in a single layer.

4. Roast for 20-30 minutes, stirring occasionally, until golden brown and crispy.

Nutrition Information (per serving):

- Calories: 150

- Protein: 8g

- Carbohydrates: 5g

- Fat: 13g

- Fiber: 2g

- Sugar: 0g

- Portion size: 1/4 cup

Indulge in these delightful dessert recipes designed to satisfy your sweet tooth while supporting your pre-diabetes management goals. Each recipe emphasizes wholesome ingredients and balanced flavors to ensure both enjoyment and nutritional benefits.

Chia Seed Pudding with Mixed Berries

Ingredients:

- 1/4 cup chia seeds
- 1 cup almond milk
- 1 tablespoon maple syrup
- 1/2 teaspoon vanilla extract
- 1 cup mixed berries (strawberries, blueberries, raspberries)

Instructions:

1. In a bowl, combine chia seeds, almond milk, maple syrup, and vanilla extract. Stir well.
2. Let the mixture sit for 15 minutes, stirring occasionally to prevent clumping.
3. Refrigerate for at least 2 hours or overnight until it reaches a pudding-like consistency.
4. Serve topped with mixed berries.

Nutrition Information (per serving):

- Calories: 180
- Protein: 5g
- Carbohydrates: 25g
- Fat: 7g
- Fiber: 10g
- Sugar: 10g
- Portion Size: 1 cup

Dark Chocolate Avocado Mousse

Ingredients:

- 2 ripe avocados
- 1/4 cup cocoa powder
- 1/4 cup maple syrup
- 1 teaspoon vanilla extract
- 1/4 cup almond milk
- Dark chocolate shavings (optional, for garnish)

Instructions:

1. Scoop out the flesh of the avocados and place in a blender or food processor.
2. Add cocoa powder, maple syrup, vanilla extract, and almond milk.

3. Blend until smooth and creamy, scraping down the sides as needed.

4. Spoon into serving dishes and refrigerate for at least 1 hour.

5. Garnish with dark chocolate shavings before serving.

Nutrition Information (per serving):

- Calories: 200

- Protein: 3g

- Carbohydrates: 25g

- Fat: 12g

- Fiber: 8g

- Sugar: 14g

- Portion Size: 1/2 cup

Baked Apples with Cinnamon

Ingredients:

- 4 apples (such as Granny Smith or Honeycrisp)

- 1 tablespoon melted coconut oil

- 1 teaspoon ground cinnamon

- 1/4 cup chopped nuts (walnuts or almonds)

Instructions:

1. Preheat the oven to 375°F (190°C).

2. Core each apple and place them in a baking dish.

3. Drizzle melted coconut oil over the apples, then sprinkle with cinnamon.

4. Bake for 25-30 minutes until apples are tender.

5. Remove from oven and sprinkle with chopped nuts before serving.

Nutrition Information (per serving):

- Calories: 150
- Protein: 2g
- Carbohydrates: 20g
- Fat: 8g
- Fiber: 5g
- Sugar: 14g
- Portion Size: 1 apple

Banana Ice Cream with Almond Butter

Ingredients:

- 4 ripe bananas, sliced and frozen
- 2 tablespoons almond butter
- 1/4 cup almond milk (optional, for creamier texture)

Instructions:

1. Place frozen banana slices in a blender or food processor.
2. Add almond butter and almond milk (if using).
3. Blend until smooth and creamy, scraping down the sides as needed.
4. Serve immediately as soft-serve or freeze for 30 minutes for a firmer texture.

Nutrition Information (per serving):

- Calories: 180
- Protein: 3g
- Carbohydrates: 30g
- Fat: 7g
- Fiber: 4g
- Sugar: 16g
- Portion Size: 1 cup

Carrot Cake Bites

Ingredients:

- 1 cup grated carrots
- 1/2 cup rolled oats
- 1/4 cup almond butter
- 1/4 cup maple syrup

- 1 teaspoon ground cinnamon
- 1/2 teaspoon ground ginger
- 1/4 cup chopped walnuts (optional, for topping)

Instructions:

1. In a food processor, combine grated carrots, rolled oats, almond butter, maple syrup, cinnamon, and ginger.
2. Pulse until well combined and mixture starts to form a dough-like consistency.
3. Roll mixture into small balls using your hands.
4. Optionally, roll each ball in chopped walnuts for coating.
5. Refrigerate for 30 minutes before serving.

Nutrition Information (per serving):

- Calories: 120
- Protein: 3g
- Carbohydrates: 15g
- Fat: 6g
- Fiber: 2g
- Sugar: 8g
- Portion Size: 2 bites

Mixed Berry Crumble

Ingredients:

- 2 cups mixed berries (strawberries, blueberries, raspberries)
- 1 tablespoon maple syrup
- 1/2 cup rolled oats
- 1/4 cup almond flour
- 2 tablespoons coconut oil, melted
- 1/4 teaspoon ground cinnamon

Instructions:

1. Preheat the oven to 350°F (175°C).
2. In a bowl, toss mixed berries with maple syrup.
3. In another bowl, combine rolled oats, almond flour, melted coconut oil, and cinnamon.
4. Spread the berries evenly in a baking dish and top with the oat mixture.
5. Bake for 25-30 minutes until the topping is golden brown and berries are bubbling.
6. Let cool slightly before serving.

Nutrition Information (per serving):

- Calories: 180
- Protein: 3g
- Carbohydrates: 25g

- Fat: 8g
- Fiber: 5g
- Sugar: 10g
- Portion Size: 1/2 cup

Coconut Macaroons

Ingredients:

- 2 cups shredded coconut (unsweetened)
- 1/2 cup coconut flour
- 1/2 cup coconut oil, melted
- 1/4 cup maple syrup
- 1 teaspoon vanilla extract
- Pinch of salt

Instructions:

1. Preheat the oven to 325°F (160°C) and line a baking sheet with parchment paper.
2. In a large bowl, mix together shredded coconut, coconut flour, melted coconut oil, maple syrup, vanilla extract, and a pinch of salt until well combined.
3. Scoop tablespoon-sized portions of the mixture and shape into small mounds or use a cookie scoop.

4. Place onto the prepared baking sheet and flatten slightly with the back of a spoon.

5. Bake for 15-18 minutes, or until the edges are golden brown.

6. Allow to cool completely on a wire rack before serving.

Nutrition Information (per serving, 2 macaroons):

- Calories: 180

- Protein: 2g

- Carbohydrates: 10g

- Fat: 15g

- Fiber: 4g

- Sugar: 6g

- Portion Size: 2 macaroons

Vegan Chocolate Chip Cookies

Ingredients:

- 1 cup almond flour

- 1/4 cup coconut oil, melted

- 1/4 cup maple syrup

- 1 teaspoon vanilla extract

- 1/2 teaspoon baking soda

- Pinch of salt

- 1/2 cup vegan chocolate chips

Instructions:

1. Preheat the oven to 350°F (175°C) and line a baking sheet with parchment paper.
2. In a bowl, mix almond flour, melted coconut oil, maple syrup, vanilla extract, baking soda, and salt until well combined.
3. Fold in vegan chocolate chips.
4. Scoop tablespoon-sized portions of dough onto the baking sheet, spacing them apart.
5. Flatten each cookie slightly with the back of a spoon.
6. Bake for 10-12 minutes, or until edges are golden brown.
7. Allow to cool on the baking sheet for 5 minutes, then transfer to a wire rack to cool completely.

Nutrition Information (per serving, 2 cookies):

- Calories: 180
- Protein: 3g
- Carbohydrates: 15g
- Fat: 12g
- Fiber: 2g
- Sugar: 10g
- Portion Size: 2 cookies

Fresh Fruit Salad with Mint

Ingredients:

- 2 cups mixed fresh fruits (such as strawberries, blueberries, kiwi, pineapple)
- 1 tablespoon fresh mint leaves, chopped
- 1 tablespoon honey or maple syrup (optional)

Instructions:

1. Wash and prepare the fruits as needed (slice strawberries, dice pineapple, etc.).
2. In a bowl, combine mixed fresh fruits and chopped mint leaves.
3. Optionally, drizzle with honey or maple syrup for added sweetness.
4. Toss gently to combine.
5. Serve immediately or refrigerate until ready to serve.

Nutrition Information (per serving):

- Calories: 100
- Protein: 1g
- Carbohydrates: 25g
- Fat: 0g
- Fiber: 4g
- Sugar: 18g

- Portion Size: 1 cup

Mango Sorbet

Ingredients:

- 2 ripe mangoes, peeled and diced
- 1/4 cup coconut milk
- 1 tablespoon honey or maple syrup (optional)
- Juice of 1 lime

Instructions:

1. Place diced mangoes in a blender or food processor.
2. Add coconut milk, honey or maple syrup (if using), and lime juice.
3. Blend until smooth and creamy.
4. Pour mixture into a shallow dish and freeze for 4-6 hours, stirring every hour to break up ice crystals.
5. Serve scoops of mango sorbet garnished with fresh mint leaves, if desired.

Nutrition Information (per serving):

- Calories: 120
- Protein: 1g
- Carbohydrates: 30g

- Fat: 1g

- Fiber: 3g

- Sugar: 25g

- Portion Size: 1/2 cup

Peanut Butter and Banana Bites

Ingredients:

- 2 bananas, sliced into rounds

- 2 tablespoons natural peanut butter

- 1/4 cup granola (choose a low-sugar variety)

Instructions:

1. Spread each banana round with a thin layer of peanut butter.

2. Sprinkle granola over half of the banana rounds.

3. Top with remaining banana rounds to form sandwiches.

4. Secure with toothpicks if desired.

5. Serve immediately or refrigerate until ready to serve.

Nutrition Information (per serving):

- Calories: 150

- Protein: 3g

- Carbohydrates: 20g

- Fat: 7g

- Fiber: 3g

- Sugar: 10g

- Portion Size: 2 bites

Roasted Pears with Honey

Ingredients:

- 4 pears, halved and cored

- 2 tablespoons honey

- 1/4 teaspoon ground cinnamon

- 1/4 cup chopped nuts (such as walnuts or almonds)

Instructions:

1. Preheat the oven to 375°F (190°C) and line a baking sheet with parchment paper.

2. Place pear halves, cut side up, on the baking sheet.

3. Drizzle honey over each pear half and sprinkle with ground cinnamon.

4. Bake for 20-25 minutes until pears are tender and caramelized.

5. Remove from oven and sprinkle with chopped nuts before serving.

Nutrition Information (per serving):

- Calories: 160
- Protein: 2g
- Carbohydrates: 30g
- Fat: 5g
- Fiber: 6g
- Sugar: 20g
- Portion Size: 1 pear half

Raw Date and Nut Bars

Ingredients:

- 1 cup Medjool dates, pitted
- 1 cup mixed nuts (such as almonds, cashews, walnuts)
- 1/4 cup shredded coconut (unsweetened)
- 1 tablespoon coconut oil, melted
- Pinch of salt

Instructions:

1. In a food processor, blend dates, mixed nuts, shredded coconut, melted coconut oil, and a pinch of salt until mixture sticks together.
2. Line a baking dish with parchment paper.
3. Press the mixture evenly into the dish.

4. Refrigerate for 1-2 hours until firm.

5. Cut into bars or squares before serving.

Nutrition Information (per serving, 1 bar):

- Calories: 180

- Protein: 4g

- Carbohydrates: 22g

- Fat: 10g

- Fiber: 4g

- Sugar: 16g

- Portion Size: 1 bar

Lemon Blueberry Muffins

Ingredients:

- 1 1/2 cups whole wheat flour

- 1/2 cup almond flour

- 1/2 cup coconut sugar

- 1 teaspoon baking powder

- 1/2 teaspoon baking soda

- Pinch of salt

- 1/4 cup coconut oil, melted

- 1 cup almond milk

- 1 tablespoon lemon zest

- 1 cup fresh or frozen blueberries

Instructions:

1. Preheat the oven to 350°F (175°C) and line a muffin tin with paper liners.
2. In a bowl, whisk together whole wheat flour, almond flour, coconut sugar, baking powder, baking soda, and salt.
3. In another bowl, mix melted coconut oil, almond milk, and lemon zest.
4. Combine wet and dry ingredients until just mixed.
5. Gently fold in blueberries.
6. Spoon batter into muffin tin, filling each cup about 3/4 full.
7. Bake for 18-20 minutes, or until a toothpick inserted into the center comes out clean.
8. Allow muffins to cool in the tin for 5 minutes before transferring to a wire rack to cool completely.

Nutrition Information (per muffin):

- Calories: 180
- Protein: 4g
- Carbohydrates: 25g
- Fat: 8g
- Fiber: 3g
- Sugar: 10g

- Portion Size: 1 muffin

Apple Cinnamon Oatmeal Bars

Ingredients:

- 2 cups rolled oats
- 1/2 cup almond flour
- 1 teaspoon ground cinnamon
- 1/4 teaspoon salt
- 1/4 cup coconut oil, melted
- 1/4 cup maple syrup
- 2 medium apples, peeled and diced
- 1/4 cup chopped walnuts (optional)

Instructions:

1. Preheat the oven to 350°F (175°C) and grease a baking dish with coconut oil.
2. In a bowl, combine rolled oats, almond flour, ground cinnamon, and salt.
3. Add melted coconut oil and maple syrup, mixing until well combined.
4. Fold in diced apples and chopped walnuts.
5. Press mixture evenly into the prepared baking dish.
6. Bake for 25-30 minutes, or until edges are golden brown.

7. Allow to cool completely before cutting into bars.

Nutrition Information (per serving, 1 bar):

- Calories: 200
- Protein: 4g
- Carbohydrates: 25g
- Fat: 9g
- Fiber: 4g
- Sugar: 10g
- Portion Size: 1 bar

Chapter 7: Smoothies

Smoothies are a delicious and convenient way to pack essential nutrients into your diet, especially when you're managing pre-diabetes. These recipes are designed to be both nutritious and satisfying, providing a variety of flavors to keep your taste buds happy. Each smoothie includes a balance of fruits, vegetables, and other wholesome ingredients to support your health goals.

Green Detox Smoothie

Ingredients:

- 1 cup spinach leaves
- 1/2 cucumber, chopped
- 1/2 green apple, cored and chopped
- 1/2 lemon, juiced
- 1/2 inch piece of ginger, peeled
- 1/2 cup coconut water
- Ice cubes (optional)

Instructions:

1. Blend all ingredients until smooth.
2. Add ice cubes if desired for a chilled texture.

Nutrition Information:

- Calories: 120
- Protein: 3g
- Carbohydrates: 28g
- Fat: 1g
- Fiber: 7g
- Sugar: 16g
- Portion Size: 1 serving

Berry Blast Smoothie

Ingredients:

- 1 cup mixed berries (strawberries, blueberries, raspberries)
- 1/2 banana
- 1/2 cup plain Greek yogurt
- 1 tbsp honey (optional)
- 1/2 cup almond milk

Instructions:

1. Combine all ingredients in a blender.
2. Blend until smooth and creamy.

Nutrition Information:

- Calories: 180

- Protein: 10g

- Carbohydrates: 32g

- Fat: 2g

- Fiber: 5g

- Sugar: 22g

- Portion Size: 1 serving

Tropical Mango Pineapple Smoothie

Ingredients:

- 1 cup frozen mango chunks

- 1/2 cup frozen pineapple chunks

- 1/2 cup coconut water

- 1/2 cup plain Greek yogurt

- 1 tbsp chia seeds (optional)

Instructions:

1. Blend mango, pineapple, coconut water, and yogurt until smooth.

2. Add chia seeds and blend for a few seconds until combined.

Nutrition Information:

- Calories: 220

- Protein: 10g

- Carbohydrates: 40g

- Fat: 3g

- Fiber: 6g

- Sugar: 32g

- Portion Size: 1 serving

Spinach and Kale Smoothie

Ingredients:

- 1 cup fresh spinach leaves

- 1 cup chopped kale leaves, stems removed

- 1/2 banana

- 1/2 cup unsweetened almond milk

- 1 tbsp almond butter

- 1 tbsp flax seeds

Instructions:

1. Blend spinach, kale, banana, almond milk, almond butter, and flax seeds until smooth.

2. Add more almond milk if needed to reach desired consistency.

Nutrition Information:

- Calories: 210

- Protein: 8g

- Carbohydrates: 21g

- Fat: 12g

- Fiber: 7g

- Sugar: 6g

- Portion Size: 1 serving

Almond Butter Banana Smoothie

Ingredients:

- 1 ripe banana

- 1 tbsp almond butter

- 1 cup unsweetened almond milk

- 1/2 tsp vanilla extract

- Ice cubes (optional)

Instructions:

1. Blend banana, almond butter, almond milk, and vanilla extract until smooth.

2. Add ice cubes if desired for a colder texture.

Nutrition Information:

- Calories: 240

- Protein: 6g

- Carbohydrates: 32g
- Fat: 10g
- Fiber: 5g
- Sugar: 17g
- Portion Size: 1 serving

Strawberry and Oat Smoothie

Ingredients:

- 1 cup fresh strawberries, hulled
- 1/2 cup rolled oats
- 1/2 cup plain Greek yogurt
- 1 tbsp honey (optional)
- 1/2 cup water or almond milk

Instructions:

1. Blend strawberries, oats, yogurt, honey, and water or almond milk until smooth.
2. Adjust consistency by adding more liquid if needed.

Nutrition Information:

- Calories: 250
- Protein: 11g
- Carbohydrates: 43g

- Fat: 4g

- Fiber: 6g

- Sugar: 14g

- Portion Size: 1 serving

Avocado and Spinach Smoothie

Ingredients:

- 1/2 ripe avocado

- 1 cup fresh spinach leaves

- 1/2 cup cucumber, chopped

- 1/2 cup pineapple chunks

- Juice of 1 lime

- 1/2 cup coconut water or water

Instructions:

1. Blend avocado, spinach, cucumber, pineapple, lime juice, and coconut water until smooth.

2. Adjust thickness with additional coconut water or water as desired.

Nutrition Information:

- Calories: 180

- Protein: 4g

- Carbohydrates: 28g
- Fat: 8g
- Fiber: 9g
- Sugar: 13g
- Portion Size: 1 serving

Blueberry and Almond Milk Smoothie

Ingredients:

- 1 cup frozen blueberries
- 1/2 banana
- 1 cup unsweetened almond milk
- 1 tbsp almond butter
- 1 tbsp honey (optional)

Instructions:

1. Blend blueberries, banana, almond milk, almond butter, and honey until smooth.
2. Adjust sweetness with more honey if desired.

Nutrition Information:

- Calories: 220
- Protein: 5g
- Carbohydrates: 35g

- Fat: 8g

- Fiber: 8g

- Sugar: 23g

- Portion Size: 1 serving

Choco-Peanut Protein Smoothie

Ingredients:

- 1 banana

- 1 tbsp cocoa powder

- 1 tbsp peanut butter

- 1 cup unsweetened almond milk

- 1 scoop vanilla protein powder (optional)

Instructions:

1. Blend banana, cocoa powder, peanut butter, almond milk, and protein powder until smooth.
2. Adjust thickness by adding more almond milk if needed.

Nutrition Information:

- Calories: 280

- Protein: 18g

- Carbohydrates: 38g

- Fat: 10g

- Fiber: 8g
- Sugar: 15g
- Portion Size: 1 serving

Kiwi and Apple Smoothie

Ingredients:

- 2 kiwis, peeled and sliced
- 1 apple, cored and chopped
- 1/2 cup spinach leaves
- 1/2 cup plain Greek yogurt
- 1/2 cup water or coconut water

Instructions:

1. Blend kiwis, apple, spinach, yogurt, and water until smooth.
2. Adjust consistency by adding more water if desired.

Nutrition Information:

- Calories: 200
- Protein: 9g
- Carbohydrates: 38g
- Fat: 3g
- Fiber: 9g
- Sugar: 25g

- Portion Size: 1 serving

Carrot and Ginger Smoothie

Ingredients:

- 1 cup carrot juice
- 1/2 inch piece of fresh ginger, peeled
- 1/2 banana
- 1/2 cup plain Greek yogurt
- Juice of 1/2 lemon

Instructions:

1. Blend carrot juice, ginger, banana, yogurt, and lemon juice until smooth.
2. Adjust flavor with more lemon juice or ginger if desired.

Nutrition Information:

- Calories: 180
- Protein: 7g
- Carbohydrates: 35g
- Fat: 2g
- Fiber: 5g
- Sugar: 20g
- Portion Size: 1 serving

Beetroot and Berry Smoothie

Ingredients:

- 1 small beetroot, peeled and diced
- 1/2 cup mixed berries (strawberries, blueberries, raspberries)
- 1/2 banana
- 1/2 cup plain Greek yogurt
- 1/2 cup water or almond milk

Instructions:

1. Blend beetroot, mixed berries, banana, yogurt, and water or almond milk until smooth.
2. Adjust consistency with more liquid if needed.

Nutrition Information:

- Calories: 220
- Protein: 10g
- Carbohydrates: 38g
- Fat: 3g
- Fiber: 8g
- Sugar: 24g
- Portion Size: 1 serving

Pineapple and Coconut Smoothie

Ingredients:

- 1 cup fresh pineapple chunks
- 1/2 cup coconut milk
- 1/2 banana
- 1/2 cup plain Greek yogurt
- 1 tbsp shredded coconut (optional)

Instructions:

1. Blend pineapple, coconut milk, banana, yogurt, and shredded coconut until smooth.
2. Garnish with additional shredded coconut if desired.

Nutrition Information:

- Calories: 250
- Protein: 8g
- Carbohydrates: 40g
- Fat: 8g
- Fiber: 5g
- Sugar: 30g
- Portion Size: 1 serving

Green Tea and Mint Smoothie

Ingredients:

- 1 cup brewed green tea, chilled
- 1/2 cup spinach leaves
- 1/2 cup fresh mint leaves
- 1/2 cup cucumber, chopped
- 1/2 banana
- Juice of 1/2 lemon

Instructions:

1. Blend green tea, spinach, mint leaves, cucumber, banana, and lemon juice until smooth.
2. Add ice cubes for a colder texture if desired.

Nutrition Information:

- Calories: 130
- Protein: 3g
- Carbohydrates: 32g
- Fat: 1g
- Fiber: 7g
- Sugar: 17g
- Portion Size: 1 serving

Citrus and Chia Seed Smoothie

Ingredients:

- 1 orange, peeled and segmented
- 1/2 cup mixed berries (strawberries, raspberries)
- 1/2 cup plain Greek yogurt
- 1 tbsp chia seeds
- 1/2 cup water or almond milk

Instructions:

1. Blend orange segments, mixed berries, yogurt, chia seeds, and water or almond milk until smooth.
2. Adjust sweetness with honey or maple syrup if desired.

Nutrition Information:

- Calories: 200
- Protein: 10g
- Carbohydrates: 30g
- Fat: 5g
- Fiber: 8g
- Sugar: 18g
- Portion Size: 1 serving

CONCLUSION

Congratulations on completing your journey through the "Pre Diabetes Vegetarian Meal Plan for Beginners"! This book was crafted with the intention of guiding you towards healthier eating habits while managing pre diabetes through delicious and nutritious vegetarian recipes.

Throughout these pages, you've discovered a diverse array of meals—from hearty breakfasts to satisfying dinners, energizing smoothies to guilt-free desserts—all designed to support your health goals without sacrificing flavor. By embracing plant-based ingredients rich in fiber, vitamins, and minerals, you've taken proactive steps towards stabilizing blood sugar levels and improving overall well-being.

Remember, this meal plan is not just about what you eat, but how you approach food as a tool for wellness. Whether you're new to vegetarianism or refining your dietary choices, the recipes provided here are meant to inspire creativity in the kitchen and empower you to make informed decisions about your nutrition.

As you continue on your journey, adapt the meal plan to suit your preferences and lifestyle, and don't hesitate to experiment with new ingredients and flavors. Consistency and mindfulness in your food choices will contribute significantly to your health journey.

We hope this book has equipped you with practical knowledge and inspiration to maintain a balanced diet that supports your journey towards better health. Remember, small changes lead to big results, and your commitment to a healthier lifestyle is a commendable step forward. Here's to your continued health and enjoyment of delicious, nourishing meals!